The Ultimate Lifting, Cardio and Motivation Bundle

By: Kelli Rae

Table of Contents

8 Weeks of Weightlifting Routines to Gain Strength and Lose Weight

42 Cardio Workouts and Other Ideas To Make Exercise Fun and Not Boring

MOTIVATION 365: Daily Inspirational Quotes to Achieve Your Goals and Dreams

8 Weeks of Weightlifting Routines to Gain Strength and Lose Weight

Introduction

This short book is intended for people who have some experience in the gym, but need a plan for their weightlifting routine. I am assuming that you have already been cleared by your doctor to undergo a weightlifting routine. I feel like there are so many people, especially women, who stay on a cardio machine for their entire workout. This isn't a bad thing, but I feel like they could maximize their results by going into the weight room. Scared? Don't be!

I have listed each exercise and the number of sets for the next 8 weeks. There are 4 to 6 routines each week, divided into various body parts. Here are some other things to keep in mind:

-Do each exercise in a controlled manner, but keep it quick.

-Take a small amount of rest in between each set.

-Each workout should take no longer than an hour.

-Don't know which weight to start with? The last few reps of the exercise should be a slight struggle. If it's too easy for you, move up in weight. If it's too difficult and you compromise form, go down in weight.

-Stay hydrated throughout the entire workout. It will help with many things, including weight loss and soreness.

Lastly, and most importantly - If you feel pain with any exercise, STOP. It's not worth an injury to do what I have written on the paper.

If you have any questions or comments about these workouts, feel free to send me an email at kelrb8@gmail.com.

ENJOY!

Chapter One - My Favorite Things

I have a simplistic mindset and you really don't need many things to get in a good workout. But here are some of my extra tools that I like to have.

Weightlifting Gloves

I like these because it protects my rings from getting scratched and tarnished. It also protects my hands. Short story - I first got these after getting some nasty calluses on my hands after boot camp one night. We were doing some bear crawls and other exercises on the floor. My hands were in bad shape after that night, and I was very thankful to get these gloves.

Bag or Backpack

Personally, I prefer backpacks over bags to carry my things. I have had my Under Armour backpack for about 8 years now, and I love it! I take it to the gym, but I also take it on the airplane, on road trips and to coffee shops. They are a little pricier, but they do last.

Headphones

This is the number one thing I need at the gym. It helps me get into "the zone" and focus. I did spend a little extra and bought Beats headphones. They stay on my head well and I do like them. I don't hear any extra music. My husband has a cheaper pair of Sony headphones, but they also work well. He just told me that they stay on his head well and the music thumps, so he is happy.

I have used other products, but these are the main things that I use on a consistent basis. Do you need any help or suggestions on picking out the correct item for your needs? Please send me an email at kelrb8@gmail.com and I will respond promptly.

Chapter Two - Week One

Legs
3x30 Alternating Lunges
3x15 DB Deadlifts

3x15 DB Squats
3x20 Jump Squats

3x15 Pistol Squats
3x50 Mountain climbers

3x15 Leg press
3x15 Hamstring curls with a stability ball

Shoulders
4x12 Seated DB Press
4x10 Seated Lateral Raises

4x20 Alternating Front DB Raises
4x15 Standing Rear Delts

3x10 Upright Rows
3x10 Burpees

3x12 Front Plate Raises
3x10 Full Range DB Circles

Back
3x15 Inverted Rows
3x25 Reverse Crunches

3x15 Pull Downs
3x25 Stability Ball Crunches

3x15 One Arm DB Rows
3x15 DB Pull Throughs

3x20 Jackknife Abs

3x15 Cable Rows
3x15 Laying Leg Lifts

Chest
4x15 DB Bench Press

3x10 Decline DB Press
3x25 Decline Crunches

3x10 Incline DB Press
3x10 Push Ups

4x15 Cable Cross-Overs
4x15 Cable Presses

3x15 Single DB Pullovers
3x50 Bicycle Cross Crunches

Arms
3x12 Candlestick Curls
3x10 Overhead DB Extensions

3x10 Super Slow DB Bicep Curls
3x10 Tricep Push Up

4x15 Straight Bar Curls
4x10 Tricep Dips

4x20 Cable Bicep Curls
4x10 Tricep Kick Backs

Chapter Three - Week Two

Legs
5x30 Alternating DB Step-ups with a Kick
5x25 Calf Raises

4x15 Leg Curls
4x15 Leg Extensions

4x20 Pistol Squats
4x30 DB Walking lunges

4x15 Leg Press
4x25 Pop Squats

Shoulders
3x15 Lateral Raises
3x10 Front Plate Raises
3x20 Hanging Abs

4x20 One arm lateral raise
4x10 One arm Shoulder Press
4x20 Your favorite ab exercise

3x15 Seated Lateral Raise
3x10 Seated Arnold Press
3x20 Reverse Crunches

4x20 Alternating Front Raises
4x20 Rear Delt Rope Pulls
1 minute plank

Back
4x15 Wide Grip pull downs
4x12 Seated Rows

3x15 Rope Pulldowns

3x15 Supermans

4x10 Cable Rows
4x10 Reverse Grip pulldowns

4x10 DB rows with a twist
4x10 DB Deadliftts

Arms
3x15 Bicep Supinated DB Curl
3x15 Overhead Tricep Extension
3x25 Crunches

3x15 Zottman Curls
3x15 DB KickBacks
3x25 Leg Lifts

3x30 Single Bicep Curls with a Cable
3x15 Straight Bar Press Downs
3x25 Hanging Leg Raises

4x15 Straight Bar Curls
4x15 Bench Dips
4x25 DB Crunches

Chest
4x15 Cable Crossovers
4x15 Push Ups

4x10 Incline Flyes
4x10 Incline DB Press

3x15 DB Pullovers with a Bridge
3x10 Pop Push Ups

3x15 Machine Chest Press
3x10 Push Ups
3x100 Stick turns

Chapter Four - Week Three

Legs
3x30 Alternating DB Step Ups
3x50 Standing Calf Raises

4x15 Leg Curls
4x15 Leg Extensions
4x10 Pop Squats

Pick an area that's about 15-20 feet long
Walking Pump Lunges - down and back is 1 set
Do 4 sets

3x20 Pistol Squats
3x20 Jump Lunges

3x20 Hack Squats
3x50 Toes Out Calf Raises

Shoulders
3x15 Rear Delt Flyes
3x10 Shrugs

4x20 One Arm Lateral Raises
4x20 One Arm Shoulder Press

3x10 Inverted Lateral Raises
3x10 Rear Delt Machine

4x10 Arnold press
4x15 Burpees

Back
4x10 Standing Straight Bar Pulldowns
4x10 Reverse Grip Pulldowns

4x16 Heavy One Arm Rows
4x10 Cable Pull Throughs

3x10 DB Deadlifts
3x15 T-Bar Rows

3x10 Supermans
3x15 Hyperextensions

Arms
4x15 Close Grip Bench Press
4x15 Skull Crushers

4x10 Bench Dips (to make it harder, put a plate on your legs)
4x10 Overhead Extension

4x10 Tricep Push Ups
4x10 Sissy Bar Curls

4x10 Seated DB Bicep Curl
1 minute Planks

4x10 Standing Cable Curls
4x10 Candlestick DB curls

Chest
3x12 Cable Crossovers
3x12 Push Ups

4x12 Incline DB Press
4x12 Decline Push Ups

3x15 Single DB Pullovers
3x10 Incline Push Ups

4x15 Machine Chest Press
4x15 Machine Chest Fly

Chapter Five - Week Four

Legs
4x20 Leg Press, wide stance
4x10 Laying Leg Curls

4x30 DB Step Ups
4x30 Jump Squats

3x20 One Legged Deadlifts
3x20 Reverse Alternating Lunges

4x10 DB Squats
4x10 Leg Extensions
4x40 Mountain Climbers

Shoulders
4x15 DB Lateral Raise
4x10 DB Shoulder Press

3x15 Upright Rows
3x10 Inverted Lateral Raise

4x15 Seated 1/2 Lateral Raise
4x15 Seated Shrugs

4x12 Shoulder Machine Press
4x10 Front Plate Raises

Back
4x10 Narrow Grip Standing Pull Downs
4x10 Pull Downs

4x10 Reverse Grip Bent Over Rows

4x10 Seated Rows
4x10 Hyperextensions

4x15 Assisted Pull Ups

Arms
4x15 Candlestick Curls
4x15 One Arm Tricep Kick Backs

3x15 Tricep Pushdowns
3x30 Mountain Climbers

4x15 Bicep Curls, keep elbows in
4x10 Sissy Bar Curls

3x10 One Handed Cable Curls
3x15 Tricep Dips, either on bench or assisted machine

Chest
4x15 Cable Crossovers, put cables at the bottom
4x15 Push Ups
4x30 Mountain Climbers

4x12 DB Bench Press
4x10 DB Pullover
4x20 Jump Squats

3x12 Incline DB Flies
3x10 Decline Push Ups
3x30 SLOW! Bicycle Cross Crunches

Chapter Six - Week Five

Legs
Do 4 sets of the following, no weights needed.

50 Squats
30 Walking Lunges
20 Jump Squats
30 Side Lunges
50 Calf Raises
30 SLOW! Bridges

Shoulders
3x20 Rear Delt Pulses
3x15 Upright Rows

3x30 Alternating Candlestick Raises
3x30 Single Side to Side Flyes

4x15 Standing DB Shoulder Press
4x15 DB Lateral Raise

3x12 Seated Arnold Press
3x30 Bicycle Cross Crunches

Back
4x30 One Arm Row with a Twist
4x20 Reverse Crunches

4x10 Wide Grip Pull Downs
4x10 Supermans

4x10 Cable Rows, pick your favorite attachment
4x30 Mountain Climbers

3x15 Hyperextensions
3x15 DB Pull Throughs

Arms/Chest
4x15 DB Bicep Curls
4x15 DB Candlestick Curls
4x30 Crunches on a Stability Ball

4x30 Concentration Curls
4x15 DB Bench Press

3x20 Dips
3x15 Overhead DB extensions

3x15 DB Flyes
3x10 Tricep Kick Backs
3x15 Pop Squats

Chapter Seven - Week Six

Legs
4x20 Walking Lunges
4x15 Pop Squats
4x20 Reverse Walking Lunges

4x15 Leg Extensions
4x10 Sumo Squats
4x15 Pop Squats

4x20 Alternating Step ups
4x20 DB DeadLifts

Shoulders
3x15 Front Plate Raise
3x15 Upright Rows
3x1 minute Planks

3x15 Seated DB Presses
3x15 Seated Rear Delts

3x15 DB Lateral Raises
3x10 Shrugs

3x15 Bent Over DB Rows
3x50 Bicycle Cross Crunches

Back
4x15 Inverted Rows
4x15 DB Deadlifts
4x20 Hanging Leg Raises

4x15 Pull Downs
4x20 Alternating side to side Pull Downs
4x20 Leg Lifts

4x10 Reverse Grip Front Pull Downs
4x15 Seated Rows

Chest
3x15 Wide Grip Push Ups
3x20 Plank Twists

3x15 DB Chest Press
3x40 Mountain Climbers

3x15 Incline DB Flyes
3x15 Decline Push Ups

3x15 Cable Cross Overs
3x12 Walkout Push up and Back
3x15 Plank Push Ups

Arms
4x15 Bicep Bar Curls
4x15 DB Candlestick Curls
4x30 Lying Stability Ball Crunches

4x30 Concentration Curls
4x20 Hand to Knee Crunches

3x20 Dips
3x15 Overhead DB extensions

3x15 Cable Push Downs
3x10 Tricep Kick Backs

90 second Plank

Chapter Eight - Week Seven

Legs
50 Mountain Climbers

4x20 Pistol Squats
4x20 One Legged Deadlifts

100 Mountain Climbers

4x12 Sumo Squats
4x20 Pop Squats

50 Walking Lunges

4x20 Alternating DB Step ups
4x20 Bench Hops

100 Walking Lunges

4x15 Hack Squats
4x20 Jump Lunges

Shoulders
4x15 Rear Delt Flyes
4x15 Upright Rows
4x20 SLOW! Russian Twists

3x15 Seated Shoulder Press
3x20 SLOW! Lying Leg Raise

3x20 Alternating Front DB Raises
3x30 Scissor Abs

4x20 Alternating DB Lateral Raises
4x15 DB Shrugs
4x20 Hanging Abs

Back
20 Plank Push Ups

3x15 Straight Bar Deadlifts
3x10 High Cable Rows

3x15 Wide Grip Pull Downs
3x15 Seated Cable Rows

3x15 Assisted Pull Ups
3x25 Jackknife Crunches

20 Plank Push Ups

Chest/Arms
3x15 DB Bench Press
3x15 DB Flyes

3x20 Seated Alternating Candlestick Curls
3x10 Push Ups

3x15 Standing Alternating DB Curls
3x15 Dips, on a bench or assisted machine
3x30 Exercise Ball Crunches

3x10 Incline DB Curls
3x15 Overhead DB Extension
3x1 minute Side Planks, 30 seconds each side

Chapter Nine - Week Eight

Legs
3x15 Burpees
3x30 Mountain Climbers
3x1 minute Sprint on Stair Stepper

3x30 Single Leg Press
3x30 Walking Lunges

4x15 Leg Extensions
4x60 second Wall Squats holding medicine ball on legs

3x15 Hamstring Curls on a Stability Ball
3x15 DB Deadlifts
3x50 Calf Raises

Shoulders/Back
4x15 Pull downs
4x15 Supermans
4x20 DB Crunches

4x15 Seated Shoulder Press
4x15 Shrugs
4x20 Hanging Leg Raises

4x10 Seated Rows
4x10 Upright Rows
4x20 Straight Leg Crunches, toes to the sky

2 minute plank

Chest
3x15 Bear Crawls
3x10 Push Ups
3x40 Bicycle Cross Crunches

3x10 Single DB Pullover
3x30 One Arm DB Fly
3x20 Reverse Crunches

3x15 DB Incline Press
3x15 DB Fly

3x15 Bench Press
3x10 Decline Push Ups
3x25 Crunches

Arms

3x12 Bottom Up 1/2 Way Curls
3x12 1/2 to Top Curls
3x25 Pop Squats

3x15 Close Grip Bench Press
3x20 Seated Alternating Bicep Curls
3x30 Mountain Climbers

3x10 Standing Cable Curls
3x15 Straight Bar Pushdowns

3x15 Skull Crushers
3x10 Candlestick Curls

Kelli Rae

42 Cardio Workouts and Other Ideas To Make Exercise Fun and Not Boring

Introduction

This short book is intended for people who need a little mix-up with their cardio routine at the gym. You may not enjoy cardio very much, or you may be short on time and not sure how to get a good workout. Let's face it - cardio can be INCREDIBLY BORING if you do the same thing all of the time, day after day. Your body can also get used to the same routine, making it harder and harder to reach any goals you may have. In part one, I have included several ideas on how to mix up your cardio routine. I have used all of these tips myself, but there are certainly other routines out these besides what I have provided. Feel free to be creative! In part two, you will find specific cardio routines that you can use at the gym so you don't even need to think about what to do. You can choose routines using a variety of equipment, from the elliptical, stairs, treadmill, bike and even no equipment at all. Feel free to use your creativity and go beyond what is in this book. The possibilities are endless!

In part three, I will give you some suggestions about other things to switch up besides doing cardio on a machine. They may be small changes, but it may be just the thing that you need.

Part One - Ideas

Phone Number

Choose a phone number. If you need help deciding on one, randomly choose a number from your phone. This will help force you to do something a little bit more challenging. If you choose all of the numbers, will you push yourself hard enough? There is a possibility of choosing "easier" numbers. Whatever you decide, these numbers are going to represent the change in levels or incline on the machine that you have chosen.

For example, let's pick the random number (888)280-3321 for a 20 minute session. After you are warmed up, do 2 minutes at level 8. Repeat this sequence 3 times, which will be for the first 3 numbers. Then do 2 minutes at level 2, 2 minutes at level 8 and so forth until you finish all of the numbers. If you choose a machine (such as a treadmill) where there are 2 items to change (level and incline), keep one of them at a constant yet challenging level, and change the other one. If you choose a phone number that has a zero, that represent level 10. If you wish to have your workout be shorter or longer than 20 minutes, adjust each number appropriately.

Tabatas

Tabatas are another type of interval training where you go hard for 20 seconds and then rest for 10 seconds. You will repeat this cycle for a total of 4 minutes and then rest for 1 minute. Repeat this again for a total of 20 minutes and you will definitely get a great workout. If you are doing the workout correctly, it should be very intense and the time will pass very quickly.

The easiest way to keep track of time is on a cardio machine of your choice. If you are doing a routine off the machine, there are a few other options. My personal favorite and preferred method is to use a timer app on a smartphone. This means you can go anywhere and not have an excuse. My favorite is called Seconds Free because you will be able to track all different kinds of intervals, including tabatas. If you would like something different, search for "tabata" or "interval" on your device and there will be several free options. Another option is to find a clock at the gym that is digital. As a last resort, you could use a clock in the gym with a seconds hand. However, make sure you are able to see it clearly and able to keep up a high same intensity.

Random Intervals

You could also choose your own intervals. For example, you could go on the elliptical, do 30 seconds of intense work followed by 45 seconds of a recovery speed for a total of 20 minutes. Or you could go to the treadmill for 20 minutes. Do an intense 20 second sprint, and then do a quick paced walk for 40 seconds. Repeat. Or you could even pick any machine and make it a game for yourself. Go as fast as you can for as long as you can. Then rest at a recovery pace for 30 seconds to a minute. Repeat. Aim to go for a specific distance or time. Do this again in a couple of weeks and try to beat your time or distance the next time you do the routine. If none of this sounds fun, use your imagination because the possibilities are endless.

If you choose this type of workout, I would recommend writing down the workout you would like to do. I suggest this because when the workout gets tough, your body may try to talk you out of a certain intensity. Do not listen! However when it's written down, it may be easier to follow because it's right there and you just have to follow it. Or you can follow one of the routines I have layed out in part two.

Pyramids

I consider this type of interval a little more advanced because you progressively do a longer amount of intensity in a short period of time. I call it a pyramid because you will start to do more intense work the longer you go in the routine.

Start with 1 minute at a low speed. Then increase your level by 8 (or an incredibly substantial amount if this isn't a challenge on your machine). Do this for 10 seconds, and then 50 seconds of your original, slow speed. Then go back up to the fast speed for 20 seconds, then 40 seconds slow. 30 seconds fast, 30 seconds slow and repeat this pattern until you do 60 seconds fast, 0 seconds slow.

If you want the workout to be even more difficult, repeat this pattern backwards (60 seconds fast, 0 slow, 50 seconds fast, 10 slow, etc).

Music Intervals

Another creative way to mix up your workouts is to use music intervals, and there are several ways you can do this. First, pick a good music station or several songs you enjoy. I think it works best to choose songs with varying tempos.

Once you're on the machine, increase or decrease your speeds depending on the tempo of the music. The song may start slow and speed up, so this is what you should do on your machine. Or, you could alternate your speeds according to the song. Go faster for one complete song, and then use the next song for recovery by going a little bit slower. Or even better, get creative and use both methods. For one song, go according to the tempo. Then for the next song, go really fast. Then for the third song, go slower and use it for recovery. Repeat.

Hopping Off Equipment

Who says you need to stay on the equipment for the entire duration? You don't - there are no rules and this is a really good way to not get bored.

There are hundreds of different options for this. One example is to pick your favorite machine in the gym. Of course, start with a warm-up and then do 5 minutes at a good pace. Then hop off and do body weight squats for a minute. Repeat this cycle for 25 minutes. If you get bored with doing squats, you could do some push-ups, mountain climbers, pop squats, jump lunges or a numerous amount of other exercises in between. It will definitely change up the pace.

Changing Equipment

Another thing you could do is change equipment. Pick your three favorite machines and do 10 minutes on each one. If you don't have a favorite, pick three at random or ask a stranger in the gym to pick. Even though you will only be on the equipment for 10 minutes at a time, make sure to keep up a good pace.

Using Weights

Another fun thing to try is cardio with weights. For safety reasons, I highly recommend sticking with the treadmill.

First, choose a pair of dumbbells and start with a light weight until you get used to doing this. From there, you have many different options. You could just hold them to the sides while you walk for extra resistance. Or, you could hold them in a static bicep curl. Or, you could even do some bicep curls. This may also be a good option if you are short on time. You could do several different upper body movements while walking and it will become a full body workout.

Part Two – Cardio Routines

Before doing any of the following routines, please make sure that you get a good warm-up. This can be as simple as 3-5 minutes walking on the treadmill at a slow, but steady pace. If you see a routine that you like under a machine that you do not have access to, please feel free to modify the routine to be appropriate for another machine.

You know your own self better than I do. You want to push yourself, but you don't want to kill yourself. These are ideas to help you as a guide, but please always check with your doctor before beginning any new exercise regimen.

Finally, when you are done with these routines, make sure to get a cool down. Please do not walk straight out of the gym immediately after finishing this routine. Doing this will not be good for your body.

Arc Trainer 1

Keep the resistance at 20 and keep a good, steady pace for the entire workout
For 3 minutes, put the incline to 6 in this order (6, 5, 4, 9, 1, 8)
1 minute, pedal backwards
3 minutes, put the incline to 5
1 minute, pedal backwards
3 minutes, incline to 4
1 minute, pedal backwards
3 minutes, incline to 9
1 minute, pedal backwards
3 minutes, incline to 1
1 minute, pedal backwards
3 minutes, incline to 8
1 minute, pedal backwards

Arc Trainer 2

Pick a random phone number
Keep the incline at 5 for entire session.
Every 3 minutes, change the resistance based on the number. You will always need to add a zero at the end.
If there is a zero in the phone number you choose, keep the same resistance as the previous number, but pedal backwards instead of forwards.
For example, for phone number 623-780-5702, start at 60, then 20, then 30, etc.

Arc Trainer 3

Start with an incline of 4 and resistance of 30
For 2 minutes, go at a good, steady pace
1 minute sprint
2 minutes, good, steady pace
1 minute sprint
Hop off and do 25 pop squats
Repeat this cycle 3 more times, increasing the incline by 1 and
the resistance by 10 each time you start a new cycle

Arc Trainer 4

Keep a steady pace throughout the workout
Minute 0-3 - incline 3-6, resistance 15-30
Min 3-5:30 - incline 0-3, resistance 30-45
Min 5:30-8 - incline 0-3, resistance 15-30
Min 8-13 - Repeat minutes 3-8
Min 13-15:30 - incline 7-10, resistance 45-60
Min 15:30-18 - max incline, resistance 30-45
Min 18-23 - Repeat minutes 13-18

AMT 1

Use medium to long strides throughout, UNLESS STATED
Minute 0-2 - resistance 0
Min 2-6 - resistance 5
Min 6-8 - resistance 5-10
Min 8-9 - resistance 10-15, stepping motion
Repeat min 6-9 two more times
Finish with 5 minutes, resistance 5-10

AMT 2

Start with 5 minutes, long strides, resistance of 10
1 minute, short strides, resistance of 15
1 minute, stepping motion, resistance of 20
Repeat this cycle 4 more times

Bike 1

Keep a good, steady pace throughout the workout UNLESS it says sprint
2 minutes, level 1
2 minutes, level 10
1 minute, level 5 SPRINT
2 minutes, level 2
2 minutes, level 9
1 minute, level 6 SPRINT
2 minutes, level 3
2 minutes, level 8
1 minute, level 7 SPRINT
2 minutes, level 4
2 minutes, level 7
1 minute, level 5 SPRINT

Bike 2

Start pedaling at level 1 for one song
Sprint for 1 minute
Increase to level 2 and pedal for one song
Go to level 1 and sprint for 1 minute
Level 3 and pedal for one song
Level 2 and sprint for 1 minute
Level 4 and pedal for one song
Level 3 and sprint for 1 minute
Level 2 and pedal for one song
Level 1 and sprint for 1 minute

Bike 3

Choose a random phone number
Every 2 minutes, change the resistance based on the number.
If there is a zero in the phone number you choose, make this
level 10.
After you have completed the entire phone number, do the
following series:
-25 squats
-25 jumping jacks
-10 push ups
-25 mountain climbers
-30 alternating lunges

Bike 4

Start at level 1 and pedal for 2 minutes
Then go to level 2 and pedal for 2 minutes
Tabata time! Machine should still be at level 2.
Sprint for 20 seconds, pedal at a slower pace for 10 seconds
Repeat this 7 more times (for a total of 4 minutes of work)
Pedal at level 1 for 1 minute
Increase to level 3
Sprint for 20 seconds, pedal at a slower pace for 10 seconds
Repeat this 7 more times (for a total of 4 minutes of work)
Pedal at level 1 for 1 minute

Bike 5

Keep all pedaling at a steady pace, but still push yourself
Start at level 2 and pedal for 3 minutes
Go to level 6 and pedal for 1 minute
Level 8 for 30 seconds
Level 10 for 30 seconds
Level 3 for 2 minutes
Level 7 for 1 minute
Level 8 for 30 seconds
Level 11 for 30 seconds
Level 2 for 3 minutes
Level 5 for 2 minutes
Level 7 for 1 minute
Level 8 for 30 seconds
Level 10 for 30 seconds
Level 2 for 2 minutes

Bike 6

Start at level 3 for 3 minutes at a steady pace
Hop off and do 50 squats
Level 4 for 3 minutes
Hop off and do 50 jumping jacks
Level 5 for 3 minutes
Hop off and do 100 calf raises
Level 6 for 3 minutes
Hop off and do 50 mountain climbers
For the next 4 minutes, keep the level at 3
Sprint for 20 minutes, pedal slower for 10 seconds
Repeat 7 more times for a total of 4 minutes
Go to level 1 and pedal for 1 minute

Elliptical 1

Begin pedaling at a moderate pace at level 3
Every 2 minutes, change from FW to BW and vice versa
Repeat this for 8 minutes
Decrease the level to 2
Sprint for 20 seconds, then go at a slower pace for 10 seconds
Repeat this 7 more times (for a total of 4 minutes of work)
Slower pace for 1 minute
Increase the level to 3
Sprint for 20 seconds, then go at a slower pace for 10 seconds
Repeat this 7 more times (for a total of 4 minutes of work)
Slower pace for 1 minute
Increase the level to 4
Sprint for 20 seconds, then go at a slower pace for 10 seconds
Repeat this 7 more times (for a total of 4 minutes of work)
Slower pace for 1 minute

Elliptical 2

Begin pedaling at a moderate pace at level 3
Maintain the moderate pace for 3 minutes
Sprint for 1 minute
Change directions and pedal backwards at a moderate pace for 1 minute
Go forwards, increase the level to 5 for 2 minutes
Sprint for 1 minute
Go backwards at a moderate pace for 1 minute
Repeat the routine two more times for a total of 27 minutes

Elliptical 3

Begin at level 1 for 1 minute at a moderate pace
Increase to level 3 for 2 minutes and increase your speed
1 minute sprint
Hop off and do 20 pop squats and 20 sumo squats
Repeat this sequence 4 times

Elliptical 4

Your choice - start at a good level for you
Pedal backwards for 1 minute at a moderate pace
Pedal forwards for 1 minute at a slightly faster pace
Double the level and sprint for 1 minute
Hop off and do 20 side to side jumps and 20 jump lunges
Repeat this sequence 4 times

Elliptical 5

(If possible) set the incline to an 8
Pick a phone number (including area code)
Every 3 minutes, change the resistance based on the phone number.
Ex: phone number you pick is 614-378-1414
Minute 5-8, resistance 6
Minute 8-11, resistance 1
Follow this pattern until all of the numbers in the phone number have been used.

Elliptical 6

Minute 0-3 - steady pace; no resistance
Min 3-6 - increase level to 3 and go at a faster, steady pace
Min 7 - 10 seconds sprint, 50 seconds steady
Min 8 - 15 seconds sprint, 45 seconds steady
Min 9 - 20 seconds sprint, 40 seconds steady
Min 10 - 25 seconds sprint, 35 seconds steady
Min 11 - 30 seconds sprint, 30 seconds steady
Min 12 - steady pace, no sprint
Increase level to 4
Min 13 - 10 seconds sprint, 50 seconds steady
Min 14 - 15 seconds sprint, 45 seconds steady
Min 15 - 20 seconds sprint, 40 seconds steady
Min 16 - 25 seconds sprint, 35 seconds steady
Min 17 - 30 seconds sprint, 30 seconds steady
Min 18-19 - steady pace, no sprint
10 minutes of abs

Stairmill 1

1 minute - Level 6
10 seconds - Level 14
50 seconds - Level 6
20 seconds - Level 14
40 seconds - Level 6
30 seconds - Level 14
30 seconds - Level 6
40 seconds - Level 14
20 seconds - Level 6
50 seconds - Level 14
10 seconds - Level 6
60 seconds - Level 14
Repeat this sequence 1 or 2 more times

Stairmill 2

Your choice - start at a moderate level for you. Please note that depending on the machine, it could calculate the level in stairs per minute or at a certain number, such as 1-20.

Minute 0-3 - moderate pace

Min 3-6 - Increase level by 1 (or by 5 stairs per minute)

Min 6-10 - Do 4 minutes of sprints. For 30 seconds, go at a moderate level and then sprint for 30 seconds at a higher level

Min 10-16 - Step sideways, 3 minutes right side then 3 minutes left side

Min 16-20 - Do another round of sprints, just like in minutes 6-10

Min 20-24 - back to a moderate pace

Stairmaster 1

Choose a set of dumbbells and begin at level 7

Go for 2 minutes at a good pace

1 minute sprint

2 minutes at a good pace

Hop off, take your dumbbells and do the following sequence -

-20 bicep curls

-20 lunges

-20 shoulder presses

Repeat this sequence two to three more times, increasing the level by 1 at the start of each new round.

Stairmaster 2

Begin at a comfortable level and step at a good pace for 5 minutes
30 second sprint
1 minute slower pace
Increase the level by 1
30 second sprint
1 minute slower pace
Hop off and do 10 push ups
Repeat this sequence until you cannot increase the levels any more

Stairmaster 3

Begin at level 6.
Go at a good pace for 4 minutes
Flip around, stand on machine backwards and go for 1 minute.
Flip back around, increase the level by 1.
Repeat this sequence 4 times

Treadmill 1

Throughout the entire workout, take nice, long strides and squeeze your glutes.
Walk at 2.5 with an incline of 0 for 3 minutes
Increase the speed to 2.8-3.0 with an incline of 10
*DO NOT hang onto the front or sides. Make sure to keep good form, but slow down the pace if it's too fast for you.

Treadmill 2

Keep the incline at 0 for the entire workout
Walk at 3.2-3.5 for 5 minutes
Tabata time!
Sprint for 20 seconds, then hop to the sides for 10 seconds.
Don't stop the speed of the treadmill
Repeat this 7 more times (for a total of 4 minutes of work)
Walk for 1 minute at 3.2-3.5
Repeat the tabatas 2 more times for a total workout of 20 minutes

Treadmill 3

I recommend some good music for this workout
Keep the incline at 2.0 for the entire workout
Walk at a medium-fast pace for one song
Jog for one song
Fast jog for one song
Walk at a medium pace for one song
For the next song, alternate between jogging and sprinting. Push yourself to your limits. Go with the flow of the music.
Walk at a medium pace for the last song

Treadmill 4

Pick a set of light to medium dumbbells.
3 minutes, hold weights to sides, walk at a medium pace, 0 incline
3 minutes, static bicep curls, walk at same pace, 3 incline
3 minutes, shoulder press, increase pace by .2, 0 incline
Hop off the treadmill and do the following:
-25 squats
-25 crunches
-25 chest press
-25 flys
Get back on the treadmill
3 minutes, hold weights to sides, walk at medium pace, 10 incline

Treadmill 5

Keep the incline at 0 for the entire workout
Minute 0-3 - walk at a steady pace
Min 3-7 - steady jog
Min 7-10 - 30 seconds sprint, 30 seconds steady jog
Min 10-14 - 15 seconds FAST and HARD sprint, 45 seconds hop to the side
Min 14-20 - steady jog

Treadmill 6

Minute 0-3 - incline 10, speed 3.4
Min 3-7:30 - incline 15, speed 3.0
Min 7:30-8 - REST (step to sides)
Min 8-11 - incline 15, speed 3.4
Min 11-11:30 - REST (step to sides)
Min 11:30-13 - incline 10, speed 4.0
Min 13-14 - REST (step to sides)
Min 14-16 - incline 10, speed 4.0
Min 16-17 - REST (step to sides)
Min 17-20 - incline 5, speed 3.5

Rowing Machine 1

Row for 500 meters at a medium, steady pace
Hop off and do 20 push ups
Row for 250 meters at a sprint
Hop off and do 50 mountain climbers
Row for 500 meters at a medium, steady pace
Hop off and do 50 fast squats
Row for 250 meters at a sprint
Hop off and do 25 pop squats

Rowing Machine 2

Row at a moderate pace for 4 minutes
Go hard for 1 minute
Hop off and do 25 pop squats
Repeat this 2 more times

Triathlon Workout

You will need an elliptical, bike, treadmill and timer.
You will do ½ mile to 1 ½ miles on each machine based on your fitness level. Choose a distance that is a challenge for you. Keep the distance the same for each piece of equipment. So if you choose ½ mile, do this for the elliptical, bike and treadmill.
Time yourself from start to finish, and record time when completed.
Do this same routine in a month with the same distance and see how much you will improve.

Multiple Machines 1

Hop on the treadmill for 15 minutes at a good walking pace (3.0-3.5) at a 2.0 incline.
Hop on the elliptical for 15 minutes, maintaining at least 140 strides per minute.
Finish with 10 minutes of abs

Multiple Machines 2

Set stairmill or stairmaster on the interval program for 20 minutes. Your choice. Push yourself throughout entire program.
Go to the treadmill and jog a mile

Multiple Machines 3

Back to the basics! Keep a good pace on each machine and do -
8 minutes elliptical
8 minutes stair master
8 minutes treadmill

Multiple Machines 4

Row for 1000 meters
Jump rope 1 minute
High knee jog 1 minute
Jumping jacks 1 minute
15 burpees
Jog on the treadmill for 1 mile
Jump rope 1 minute
Mountain climbers 1 minute
15 pop squats
Elliptical for 10 minutes - keep a good pace
Jump rope 1 minute
100 squats

Multiple Machines 5

Jog for 2 miles
Stairs for 5 minutes at a good pace
Elliptical for 10 minutes, level 10
Treadmill for 10 minutes, sprinting for 30 seconds and resting for 30 seconds
Walk at a good pace for 5 minutes

Multiple Machines 6

Start on the treadmill and do the following -
4 minutes, 10 incline, 3.0 speed
2 minutes, 5 incline, 3.5 speed
Put the incline to 0
For the next 4 minutes, do the following -
30 seconds sprint
30 seconds rest
Repeat sprinting cycle 3 more times
Go to the elliptical and go at a good pace for 8 minutes
Finish on the stairmill and go at a good pace for 8 minutes

No Machines 1

2 sets:
-50 jumping jacks

-50 toe taps
-50 body weight squats
-50 calf raises
-50 total alternating lunges
-50 one legged deadlifts
-50 mountain climbers
-50 total step ups, alternating

No Machines 2

50 jumping jacks
10 push ups
10 burpees
50 pop squats
100 mountain climbers
1 minute air jump rope
Repeat 2 more times
Finish with a jog for about 5 minutes. No need to time - just estimate.

No Machines 3

Tabata time!
Do the following exercises for 20 seconds, and rest in between each exercise for 10 seconds.
-alternating lunges
-pop squats
-mountain climbers
-jumping jacks
-leap frogs
-jump lunges
-jog in place
-burpees
Rest for 1 minute
Repeat cycle 3 more times

No Machines 4

FINAL CHALLENGE!
Start with a light jog for about 5 minutes
10 push ups
20 side to side jumps
30 skaters
40 pop squats
50 crunches
60 jumping jacks
70 mountain climbers
80 alternating lunges (total)
90 high knee jog
100 squats
Finish with burpees to failure

Part Three – Other Ideas

I always tell people that a gym is great, but you don't NEED one to be healthy and fit. Here are some other ideas for exercise. You may hate the gym, can't make it one day, can't afford it, or just want something different to do for a workout. Whatever the reason may be, here are some ideas for you to try.

Go Outside
The possibilities are limitless. You can talk a walk by yourself or do one of the "no-machine" cardio routines I included in this book. Or call up a friend and enjoy a nice walk. Mix it up and have fun!

Join a Class
There are many options available for this. If you do have a gym membership, there may be classes offered for no extra charge beyond your monthly dues. If you don't have one, don't worry! There are other facilities that offer classes, anywhere from CrossFit, to hot yoga and Zumba. If you have a limited budget, go online and visit Groupon. Depending on your area, there may be hundreds of options for you at a very reasonable cost. Be daring and who knows if you will find something that you really love.

Hire a Personal Trainer
This may put some "spice" back into your workouts. Some gyms may even offer some free sessions. They tend to be on the expensive side. However, if you are able to hire one on a consistent basis, it could help with your goals. You will know that you need to meet with them on X date, so you may work a little bit harder.

Share a Trainer
Maybe you like the idea of a personal trainer, but you cannot afford it. Find out if you can share the hour with a few

friends in a group session. Believe me, you will still get a good workout and it will be a lot of fun!

Find a Gym Buddy

I'm sure there are people at your gym that may in your same situation. Working out with someone else with similar goals can be encouraging and a lot of fun. Talk to people at the gym or find someone on social media to meet up with. You'll be able to push each other and reach goals even faster.

Non-Workout Ideas

So after reading this, you may feel like you mix up your cardio pretty well. However, maybe you're still bored and need something fresh. There are several different things that you can do to make you look forward to the gym and your next cardio workout.

It is essential that you find a type of exercise that you enjoy. It's definitely not mandatory to join a gym and do cardio as part of your routine. If the thought of getting on a cardio machine or even going to a gym makes you want to throw up, then don't do it. The point is just to exercise for health. There are numerous other ways to be active, and you should definitely find something that you enjoy and makes you happy.

New music - It is time to change up your music if you are able to know what song is coming up next. Just by changing your music, you may look forward to your next workout.

YouTube - do you have free wi-fi at the gym or sufficient data to watch videos? Make sure to still keep up the intensity, but there are hundreds of thousands of hours on so many topics on there to watch.

New outfit, shoes or bag

Yummy healthy meal afterwards you can look forward to - I used to make healthy protein ice cream, and it would "make" while I was at the gym. When a routine was tough, I'd think about my "ice cream" and it seemed easier.

MOTIVATION 365 Daily Inspirational Quotes to Achieve Your Goals and Dreams

Introduction

It was always a dream of mine to own my own business and do what I wanted for a living. Although I never really figured out exactly what I wanted to do for a career, I knew that I didn't want to work for anyone else. In my youth, whenever people would ask me what I wanted to be when I grew up, I always changed my mind—but one thing remained constant: it was never a desk job. To me, a typical desk job is the equivalent of working in shackles and having no freedom. I didn't want that kind of life.

Fast forward two years after college, and that's exactly where I ended up - at a desk job. I remember the very first day, when my boss showed me my desk and I felt like I was going to prison. I still didn't want that at all, but I really didn't know what else to do. These feelings would continue for the next several years. I would come home from work stressed and in tears, and I knew something had to change.

Finally in February 2013, enough was enough. I didn't care how much money I was making in corporate America. I had to be happy. So I decided to turn my hobby of reselling things into a full-time business. I had always enjoyed couponing and finding deals, so why not make that into a career?

It has not been an easy road, but I have since created my own LLC and continue to work hard at growing my business. Although I still have a desk, I feel like I have more freedom because I can work when I want instead of following someone else's schedule. No more prison for me! I enjoy my work, and I am my own boss. I put in more hours now, but I wouldn't have it any other way.

If you are reading this book, maybe you are in the same situation that I was. Maybe you absolutely hate your job, but you don't know what else to do or lack the motivation. That's where this book comes in. I have personally selected and compiled 365 quotes that will hopefully inspire you to make a change and do something that you enjoy. Each of these quotes have special meaning to me. Life is way too short to do something that you hate. The journey will not be easy, but it will be worth it.

How you read this book is up to you. You could read one quote every morning and spend a few moments thinking about it before starting your day. You could read an entire page (or several pages) all at once on a day when you're feeling down about life. You could even cut the quotes out and tape them around your house for constant reminders to work hard and follow your dreams. Use your imagination!

Kelli Rae

Motivation 365

1

Success is doing what you want to do, when you want, where you want, with whom you want, as much as you want.
-Anthony Robbins, life coach/self-help author

2

Life is about making an impact, not making an income.
-Kevin Kruse, NY Times bestselling author

3

You may have to fight a battle more than once to win it.
-Margaret Thatcher, former Prime Minister of the United Kingdom

4

Wealth is enjoying what we already have, not getting more of what we think will make us happy.
-Peter McWilliams, American self-help author

5

I would rather fail in an attempt at something new and uncharted than safely succeed in a repeat of something I have done.
-A. E. Hotchner, American novelist

6
Man was designed for accomplishment, engineered for success, and endowed with the seeds of greatness.
-Zig Ziglar, American author/motivational speaker

7
It's not about ideas. It's about making ideas happen.
-Scott Belsky, co-founder of Behance

8
It is not easy to find happiness in ourselves, and it is not possible to find it elsewhere.
-Agnes Repplier, American essayist

9
You can't build a reputation on what you're going to do.
-Henry Ford, American industrialist

10
Be miserable. Or motivate yourself. Whatever has to be done, it's always your choice. **-Wayne Dyer, American self-help author**

11
The greatest mistake you can make in life is to continually be afraid you will make one.
-Elbert Hubbard, American writer

12
Never give up on something that you can't go a day without thinking about.
-Sir Winston Churchill, British politician, Prime Minister

13
Vision gives you the impulse to make the picture your own.
-Robert Collier, American author of self-help books

14
I wanted to change the world. But I have found that the only thing one can be sure of changing is oneself.
-Aldous Huxley, English philosopher

15
Toughness is in the soul and spirit, not in muscles.
-Alex Karras, football player

16
When I was 5 years old, my mother always told me that happiness was the key to life. When I went to school, they asked me what I wanted to be when I grew up. I wrote down 'happy'. They told me I didn't understand the assignment, and I told them they didn't understand life.
-John Lennon, English singer/songwriter

17

More important than talent, strength, or knowledge is the ability to laugh at yourself and enjoy the pursuit of your dreams.

-Amy Grant, singer/songwriter

18

Perseverance is the hard work you do after you get tired of doing the hard work you already did.

-Newt Gingrich, American politician

19

What makes something special is not just what you have to gain, but what you feel there is to lose.

-Andre Agassi, retired American professional tennis player

20

Life itself is a privilege, but to live life to the fullest- well, that is a choice.

-Andy Andrews, American author

21

Do what you can, where you are, with what you have.

-Theodore Roosevelt, 26th U.S. President

22
To be upset over what you don't have is to waste what you do have.
-Ken Keyes, American personal growth author

23
First, have a definite, clear practical ideal; a goal, an objective. Second, have the necessary means to achieve your ends; wisdom, money, materials, and methods. Third, adjust all your means to that end.
-Aristotle, Greek philosopher

24
Keep digging. Nobody said it's going to be easy. You have to dig into yourself. Think about your family, think about the journey itself. Think in the moment.
-Meb Keflezighi, 2004 Olympic silver medalist (marathon)

25
I feel the most important requirement to success is learning to overcome failure. You must learn to tolerate it, but never accept it.
-Reggie Jackson, retired baseball player

26
In life, as in football, you won't go far unless you know where the goalposts are.
-Arnold Glasow, American author

27
Ability is what you are capable of doing. Motivation determines what you do. Attitude determines how well you do it.
-Lou Holtz, college football analyst

28
The question isn't who is going to let me; it's who is going to stop me.
-Ayn Rand, Russian-American novelist

29
Opportunity rarely knocks on your door. Knock rather on opportunity's door if you ardently wish to enter.
-B. C. Forbes, Scottish-born American financial journalist

30
Success is a journey...not a destination.
-Ben Sweetland, author

31
All things are possible until they are proved impossible and even the impossible may only be so, as of now.
-Pearl S. Buck, American writer/novelist

32
The best way to predict the future is to invent it.
-Alan Kay, American computer scientist

33

I always did something I was a little not ready to do. I think that's how you grow. When there's that moment of 'Wow, I'm not really sure I can do this,' and you push through those moments, that's when you have a breakthrough.
-Marissa Mayer, CEO of Yahoo

34

Twenty years from now you will be more disappointed by the things that you didn't do than by the ones you did do, so throw off the bowlines, sail away from safe harbor, catch the trade winds in your sails. Explore, Dream, Discover.
-Mark Twain, American author/humorist

35

I think the foremost quality – there's no success without it – is really loving what you do. If you love it, you do it well, and there's no success if you don't do well what you're working at.
-Malcolm Forbes, American entrepreneur

36

Commitment leads to action. Action brings your dream closer.
-Marcia Wieder, founder and CEO of Dream University

37

Risk more than others think is safe. Dream more than others think is practical.
-Howard Schultz, CEO of Starbucks

38
I have looked in the mirror every morning and asked myself: 'If today were the last day of my life, would I want to do what I am about to do today?' And whenever the answer has been 'No' for too many days in a row, I know I need to change something.
-Steve Jobs, American entrepreneur/inventor

39
To gain more abundance a person needs more skills and needs to be more creative and cooperative.
-Robert Kiyosaki, American investor

40
You don't become enormously successful without encountering some really interesting problems.
-Mark Victor Hansen, American motivational speaker/author

41
Be fearless. Have the courage to take risks. Go where there are no guarantees. Get out of your comfort zone even if it means being uncomfortable. The road less traveled is sometimes fraught with barricades, bumps, and uncharted terrain. But it is on that road where your character is truly tested. Have the courage to accept that you're not perfect, nothing is and no one is — and that's OK.
-Katie Couric, American journalist/author

42
The only people who never fail are those who never try.
-Ilka Chase, American actress and novelist

43
In order to succeed, your desire for success should be greater than your fear of failure. **-Bill Cosby, American stand-up comedian**

44
Champions keep playing until they get it right.
-Billie Jean King, retired American tennis player

45
The only way to find the limits of the possible is by going beyond them to the impossible.
-Arthur C. Clarke, British science fiction writer

46
Exceed expectations. We are not driven to do extraordinary things, but to do ordinary things extraordinarily well.
-Charles Gore, bishop/theologian

47
Timing, perseverance, and ten years of trying will eventually make you look like an overnight success.
-Biz Stone, co-founder of Twitter

48
You are what you think. You are what you go for. You are what you do.
-Bob Richards, Olympic athlete

49
The men who have succeeded are men who have chosen one line and stuck to it.
-Andrew Carnegie, Scottish-American industrialist

50
Just because Fate doesn't deal you the right cards, it doesn't mean you should give up. It just means you have to play the cards you get to their maximum potential.
-Les Brown, motivational speaker and former politician

51
If you just work on stuff that you like and you're passionate about, you don't have to have a master plan with how things will play out.
-Mark Zuckerberg, founder of Facebook

52
Take the first step in faith. You don't have to see the whole staircase, just take the first step.
-Dr. Martin Luther King, Jr., activist/humanitarian

53
If you want to know your past, look into your present conditions. If you want to know your future, look into your present actions.
-Buddhist Saying

54
Life shrinks or expands in proportion to one's courage.
-Anais Nin, author

55
Successful people tend to become more successful because they are always thinking about their successes.
-Brian Tracy, American author/motivational speaker

56
With ordinary talents and extraordinary perseverance, all things are attainable.
-Sir Thomas Fowell Buxton, English member of Parliament

57
Don't be afraid to give up the good to go for the great.
-John D. Rockefeller, American business magnate/philanthropist

58
Change is the law of life. And those who look only to the past or present are certain to miss the future.
-John F Kennedy, 35th U.S. President

59
Your habits will determine your quality of life. It's so hard when contemplated in advance, and so easy when you just do it.
-Robert M. Pirsig, American writer/philosopher

60
Work for the fun of it, and the money will arrive some day.
-Ronnie Milsap, American country music singer

61
Whatever you can do, or dream you can, begin it. Boldness has genius, power and magic in it.
-Johann Wolfgang von Goethe, German writer

62
Take up one idea. Make that one idea your life--think of it, dream of it, live on that idea. Let the brain, muscles, nerves, every part of your body, be full of that idea, and just leave every other idea alone. This is the way to success.
-Swami Vivekananda, Indian Hindu monk

63

Happiness is a butterfly, which when pursued, is always beyond your grasp, but which, if you will sit down quietly, may alight upon you.
-Nathaniel Hawthorne, American author

64

I have never run into a guy who could win at the top level in anything today and didn't have the right attitude, didn't give it everything he had, at least while he was doing it; wasn't prepared and didn't have the whole program worked out.
-Ted Turner, founder of CNN/philanthropist

65

Never let a day pass that will make you say, "I will do better tomorrow".
-Brigham Young, American leader

66

Nothing splendid has ever been achieved except by those who dared believe that something inside of them was superior to circumstance.
-Bruce Barton, American author/politician

67

Nothing in the world can take the place of persistence. Talent will not; nothing is more common than unsuccessful men with talent. Genius will not; unrewarded genius is almost a proverb ... Persistence and determination alone are omnipotent.
-Calvin Coolidge, 30th U.S. President

68
The way to get started is to quit talking and begin doing.
-Walt Disney, co-founder of the Walt Disney Company.

69
Failure is the tuition you pay for success.
-Walter Brunell, author

70
Happiness is an attitude. We either make ourselves miserable, or happy and strong. The amount of work is the same.
-Carlos Castaneda, American author

71
If you always put limit on everything you do, physical or anything else. It will spread into your work and into your life. There are no limits. There are only plateaus, and you must not stay there, you must go beyond them.
-Bruce Lee, actor/martial arts expert

72
Experience taught me a few things. One is to listen to your gut, no matter how good something sounds on paper. The second is that you're generally better off sticking with what you know. And the third is that sometimes your best investments are the ones you don't make.
-Donald Trump, American business magnate

73
I wouldn't say anything is impossible. I think that everything is possible as long as you put your mind to it and put the work and time into it.
-Michael Phelps, multiple Olympic gold medalist (swimming)

74
The distance between insanity and genius is measured only by success.
-Bruce Feirstein, American screenwriter/humorist

75
Falling in life is inevitable - staying down is optional
-Carrie Johnson, 2 time Olympic kayaker

76
How you think about a problem is more important than the problem itself - so always think positively.
-Norman Vincent Peale, author/minister

77
Work as though you would live forever, and live as though you would die today.
-Og Mandino, American author

78
You will never find time for anything. If you want time, you must make it.
-Charles Buxton, English philanthropist

79
Never continue in a job you don't enjoy. If you're happy in what you're doing, you'll like yourself, you'll have inner peace. And if you have that, along with physical health, you will have had more success than you could possibly have imagined.
-Johnny Carson, American television host

80
When you find an idea that you just can't stop thinking about, that's probably a good one to pursue.
-Josh James, founder and CEO of Omniture

81
One fails forward toward success.
-Charles F. Kettering, American inventor

82
Like what you do. If you don't like it, do something else.
-Paul Harvey, American radio broadcaster

83

The secret to productive goal setting is in establishing clearly defined goals, writing them down and then focusing on them several times a day with words, pictures and emotions as if we've already achieved them.
-Denis Waitley, American motivational speaker

84

A dream doesn't become reality through magic; it takes sweat, determination and hard work.
-Colin Powell, American statesman

85

If you dream and you allow yourself to dream you can do anything.
-Clara Hughes, multiple Olympic medalist in cycling and speed skating

86

The reward of a thing well done is to have done it.
-Ralph Waldo Emerson, 19th century American essayist

87

If you want to reach a goal, you must see yourself reaching it in your own mind before you actually arrive at your goal.
-Zig Ziglar, American author/motivational speaker

88
Life is full of small victories along the way. If you ever start feeling, 'I've achieved everything I'm going to achieve. I've mastered this. I've mastered my life,' I think you cease to live. You stop caring. You stop striving. I think that's what living is really all about.
-Condoleezza Rice, 66th United States Secretary of State

89
Determination and perseverance move the world; thinking that others will do it for you is a sure way to fail.
-Marva Collins, American educator

90
Four steps to achievement: Plan purposefully. Prepare prayerfully. Proceed positively. Pursue persistently.
-William Arthur Ward, writer

91
It does not matter how slowly you go as long as you do not stop.
-Confucius, philosopher

92
Efforts and courage are not enough without purpose and direction.
-John F. Kennedy, 35th U.S. President

93
Most of the important things in the world have been accomplished by people who have kept on trying when there seemed to be no help at all.
-Dale Carnegie, American writer

94
Don't aim for success if you want it; just do what you love and believe in, and it will come naturally.
-David Frost, English journalist

95
Nothing is stronger than habit.
-Ovid, Roman poet

96
Only put off until tomorrow what you are willing to die having left undone.
-Pablo Picasso, Spanish artist

97
The important thing is not being afraid to take a chance. Remember, the greatest failure is to not try. Once you find something you love to do, be the best at doing it.
-Debbi Fields, founder of Mrs. Fields Cookies

98
Setting a goal is not the main thing. It is deciding how you will go about achieving it and staying with that plan.
-Tom Landry, American football player/coach

99
The reason most people never reach their goals is that they don't define them, or ever seriously consider them as believable or achievable. Winners can tell you where they are going, what they plan to do along the way, and who will be sharing the adventure with them.
-Denis Waitley, American motivational speaker

100
The man who does not work for the love of work but only for money is not likely to make money nor find much fun in life.
-Charles Schwab, American businessman

101
Once you choose hope, anything's possible.
-Christopher Reeve, actor/author

102
Keep your fears to yourself, but share your courage with others.
-Robert Louis Stevenson, Scottish novelist

103

Don't wait for someone else to make your life terrific. That's your job.
-Unknown

104

A man can be as great as he wants to be. If you believe in yourself and have the courage, the determination, the dedication, the competitive drive and if you are willing to sacrifice the little things in life and pay the price for the things that are worthwhile, it can be done.
-Vince Lombardi, head coach of the Green Bay Packers (1959-1967)

105

There may be people that have more talent than you, but there's no excuse for anyone to work harder than you do.
-Derek Jeter, retired American baseball player

106

Don't be intimidated by what you don't know. That can be your greatest strength and ensure that you do things differently from everyone else.
-Sara Blakely, founder of Spanx

107

I think the one lesson I have learned is that there is no substitute for paying attention. **-Diane Sawyer, American journalist**

108

You just have to be yourself and go full with confidence and be courageous.
-Gabrielle Douglas, gymnast and Olympic gold medalist

109

As long as you're going to be thinking anyway, think big.
-Donald Trump, American business magnate

110

Never let your memories be greater than your dreams.
-Doug Ivester, former Chairman and CEO of Coca-Cola Company

111

Start by doing what's necessary, then what's possible, and suddenly you are doing the impossible.
-St. Francis of Assisi, Italian Catholic preacher

112

People with goals succeed because they know where they are going... It's as simple as that.
-Earl Nightingale, English social reformer

113

The mind is everything. What you think you become.
-Buddha

114

To be successful, you must decide exactly what you want to accomplish, then resolve to pay the price to get it.
-Bunker Hunt, American oil company executive

115

There is no point at which you can say, "Well I am successful now, I might as well relax". - **-Carrie Fisher, American actress**

116

You'll never do a whole lot unless you're brave enough to try.
-Dolly Parton, singer/songwriter

117

Leadership is the capacity to translate vision into reality.
-Warren Bennis, American scholar

118

The secret of success is this: there is no secret to success.
-Elbert Hubbard, American writer

119

It is our attitude at the beginning of a difficult task which, more than anything else, will affect its successful outcome.
-William James, American philosopher/psychologist

120
It is not fair to ask of others what you are unwilling to do yourself.
-Eleanor Roosevelt, politician/activist

121
Just don't give up trying to do what you really want to do. Where there is love and inspiration, I don't think you can go wrong.
-Ella Fitzgerald, American jazz singer

122
If you genuinely want something, don't wait for it - teach yourself to be impatient.
-Gurbaksh Chahal, Internet entrepreneur/writer

123
Don't say you don't have enough time. You have exactly the same number of hours per day that were given to Helen Keller, Pasteur, Michaelangelo, Mother Teresea, Leonardo da Vinci, Thomas Jefferson, and Albert Einstein.
-H. Jackson Brown Jr., American author

124
I work really hard at trying to see the big picture and not getting stuck in ego. I believe we're all put on this planet for a purpose, and we all have a different purpose... When you connect with that love and that compassion, that's when everything unfolds.
-Ellen DeGeneres, comedian/philanthropist

125
There are two ways of meeting difficulties: you can alter the difficulties, or you can alter yourself to meet the difficulties.
-Phyllis Bottoms, British novelist

126
There is no substitute for hard work.
-Thomas Edison, American inventor/businessman

127
To uncover your true potential you must first find your own limits and then you have to have the courage to blow past them.
-Picabo Street, Olympic gold medalist (skiing)

128
Make the best use of what is in your power, and take the rest as it happens.
-Epictetus, Greek philosopher

129
Success is the sum of small efforts repeated day in and day out.
-Robert Collier, American author of self-help books

130
If we succeed, it will not be because of what we have, but it will be because of what we are; not because of what we own, but, rather because of what we believe.
-Lyndon B Johnson, 36th U.S. President

131
And the trouble is, if you don't risk anything, you risk even more.
-Erica Jong, American author

132
Everything begins with a decision. Then, we have to manage that decision for the rest of your life.
-John C. Maxwell, American author/speaker

133
Many people dream of success. To me success can only be achieved through repeated failure and introspection.
-Soichiro Honda, Japanese engineer/industrialist

134
It is not the size of a man but the size of his heart that matters.
-Evander Holyfield, retired American boxer

135
I am a great believer in luck, and l find that the harder I work the more luck I have. **-Thomas Jefferson, American Founding Father, 3rd U.S. President**

136
For all of the most important things, the timing always sucks. Waiting for a good time to quit your job? The stars will never align and the traffic lights of life will never all be green at the same time. The universe doesn't conspire against you, but it doesn't go out of its way to line up the pins either. Conditions are never perfect. "Someday" is a disease that will take your dreams to the grave with you. Pro and con lists are just as bad. If it's important to you and you want to do it "eventually," just do it and correct course along the way.
-Timothy Ferriss, author of The 4-Hour Work Week

137
You never know what you are capable of until you decide what you want and then you just have to go for it.
-Fantasia Barrino, actress/singer

138
I am not a has-been. I am a will be.
-Lauren Bacall, actress

139
Live daringly, boldly, fearlessly. Taste the relish to be found in competition - in having put forth the best within you.
-Henry J. Kaiser, American industrialist/became known as the father of modern American shipbuilding

140
The thing always happens that you really believe in; and the belief in a thing makes it happen.
-Frank Lloyd Wright, American architect/educator

141
Don't let the opinions of the average man sway you. Dream, and he thinks you're crazy. Succeed, and he thinks you're lucky. Acquire wealth, and he thinks you're greedy. Pay no attention. He simply doesn't understand.
-Robert G. Allen, author

142
If there is no struggle, there is no progress.
-Frederick Douglass, African-American social reformer

143
Light tomorrow with today.
-Elizabeth Barrett Browning, English poet

144
We tend to forget that happiness doesn't come as a result of getting something we don't have, but rather of recognizing and appreciating what we do have.
-Frederick Koenig, German inventor

145
What you lack in talent can be made up with desire, hustle, and giving 110 percent all the time.
-Don Zimmer, former American baseball player/coach

146
People are always blaming circumstances for what they are. I don't believe in circumstances. The people who get ahead in this world are the people who get up and look for the circumstances they want, and if they can't find them, make them.
-George Bernard Shaw, Irish playwright

147
The groundwork of all happiness is health.
-Leigh Hunt, English writer

148
The things you want are always possible; it is just that the way to get them is not always apparent. The only real obstacle in your path to a fulfilling life is you, and that can be a considerable obstacle because you carry the baggage of insecurities and past experience. **-Les Brown, motivational speaker and former politician**

149
The past doesn't define you, your present does. It's okay to create a vision of the future because it affects your behavior in the "now," but don't dwell on past mistakes. Learn from them and focus those lessons in the moment. That's where change can really happen.
-Jillian Michaels, celebrity trainer

150
Nothing is easy to the unwilling.
-Thomas Fuller, English churchman/historian

151
The only failure one should fear, is not hugging to the purpose they see as best.
-George Eliot, English writer/pen name of Mary Ann Evans

152
You've got to get up every morning with determination if you're going to go to bed with satisfaction.
-George Horace Lorimer, American journalist and author

153
The starting point of all achievement is DESIRE. Keep this constantly in mind. Weak desire brings weak results, just as a small fire makes a small amount of heat.
-Napoleon Hill, American author

154
The major value in life is not what you get. The major value in life is what you become. **-Jim Rohn, American entrepreneur**

155
Dreaming, after all, is a form of planning.
-Gloria Steinem, American journalist/activist

156
Each of us has a fire in our hearts for something. It's our goal in life to find it and keep it lit.
-Mary Lou Retton, Olympic gold medalist (gymnastics)

157
Whatever course you decide upon, there is always someone to tell you that you are wrong. There are always difficulties arising which tempt you to believe that your critics are right. To map out a course of action and follow it to an end requires courage.
-Ralph Waldo Emerson, 19th century American essayist

158
Life is what we make it, always has been, always will be.
-Grandma Moses, American folk artist

159
Opportunity is just success looking for a place to happen.
-Greg Hickman, American businessman, online entrepreneur

160
I am not a product of my circumstances. I am a product of my decisions.
-Stephen Covey, American author

161
Always remember, you have within you the strength, the patience, and the passion to reach for the stars to change the world.
-Harriet Tubman, African-American humanitarian

162
One of the lessons that I grew up with was to always stay true to yourself and never let what somebody else says distract you from your goals. And so when I hear about negative and false attacks, I really don't invest any energy in them, because I know who I am.
-Michelle Obama, American lawyer/writer

163

The critical ingredient is getting off your butt and doing something. It's as simple as that. A lot of people have ideas, but there are few who decide to do something about them now. Not tomorrow. Not next week. But today. The true entrepreneur is a doer, not a dreamer.
-Nolan Bushnell, founder of Atari and Chuck-E-Cheese's

164

The whole secret of a successful life is to find out what is one's destiny to do, and then do it.
-Henry Ford, American industrialist

165

Dreams are lovely. But they are just dreams. Fleeting, ephemeral, pretty. But dreams do not come true just because you dream them. It's hard work that makes things happen. It's hard work that creates change.
-Shonda Rhimes, screenwriter

166

It is the heart that makes a man rich. He is rich according to what he is, not according to what he has.
-Henry Ward Beecher, American social reformer

167
I cannot give you the formula for success, but I can give you the formula for failure - which is: Try to please everybody.
-Herbert Bayard Swope, American journalist

168
Talent is only the starting point.
-Irving Berlin, Russian-born Jewish-American composer/lyricist

169
I attribute my success to this: I never gave or took any excuse.
-Florence Nightingale, English reformer/statistician

170
Only he who can see the invisible can do the impossible.
-Frank L Gaines, former mayor

171
Achievement is largely the product of steadily raising one's levels of aspirations and expectations.
-Jack Nicklaus, retired golfer

172
If you set your goals ridiculously high and it's a failure, you will fail above everyone else's success.
-James Cameron, Canadian film director/producer

173
Nothing could be worse than the fear that one had given up too soon, and left one unexpended effort that might have saved the world.
-Jane Addams, leader in womens suffrage and world peace

174
You may be disappointed if you fail, but you are doomed if you don't try.
-Beverly Sills, American operatic soprano

175
The price of doing the same old thing is far higher than the price of change.
-Bill Clinton, 42ⁿᵈ U.S. President

176
Life isn't about finding yourself. Life is about creating yourself.
-George Bernard Shaw, Irish playwright

177
Identity is a prison you can never escape, but the way to redeem your past is not to run from it, but to try to understand it, and use it as a foundation to grow.
-Jay-Z, American rapper and record producer

178
We must embrace pain and burn it as fuel for our journey.
-Kenji Miyazawa, Japanese poet

179
It's important to push yourself further than you think you can go each and every day - as that is what separates the good from the great.
-Kerri Strug, retired gymnast

180
I knew that if I failed I wouldn't regret that, but I knew the one thing I might regret is not trying.
-Jeff Bezos, CEO and founder of Amazon

181
We all have dreams. But in order to make dreams come into reality, it takes an awful lot of determination, dedication, self discipline, and effort.
-Jesse Owens, four-time Olympic gold medalist (track and field)

182

Failure is all a matter of perspective. Think of all the people you admire. I guarantee you they all failed at one time or another. The key is to recognize setbacks for what they really are—entry points for learning, not validation that you aren't good enough. After a disappointment analyze your actions, get feedback from friends, and take inventory of what you could do better next time. This type of self-reflection and improvement will ultimately make success inevitable. **-Jillian Michaels, celebrity trainer**

183

The impossible is often the untried.
-Jim Goodwin, Irish soccer player

184

Successful people do what unsuccessful people are not willing to do. Don't wish it were easier, wish you were better.
-Jim Rohn, American entrepreneur

185

A good plan violently executed right now is far better than a perfect plan executed next week.
-George Patton, US Army general

186

99% of the failures come from people who have the habit of making excuses.
-George Washington Carver, American botanist/inventor

187

In my experience, there is only one motivation, and that is desire. No reasons or principle contain it or stand against it.
-Jane Smiley, American novelist

188

Do you want to be safe and good, or do you want to take a chance and be great?
-Jimmy Johnson, American football broadcaster

189

You don't get to choose how you're going to die, or when. You can only decide how you're going to live now.
-Joan Baez, American folk singer/songwriter

190

You can't connect the dots looking forward; you can only connect them looking backwards. So you have to trust that the dots will somehow connect in your future. You have to trust in something--your gut, destiny, life, karma, whatever. This approach has never let me down, and it has made all the difference in my life.
-Steve Jobs, American entrepreneur/inventor

191

Success without honor is an unseasoned dish; it will satisfy your hunger, but it won't taste good.
-Joe Paterno, American college football player/coach

192

Just trust yourself, then you will know how to live.
-Johann Wolfgang Von Goethe, German writer

193

Success is ... knowing your purpose in life, growing to reach your maximum potential, and sowing seeds that benefit others.
-John C. Maxwell, American author/speaker

194

The common denominator for success is work.
-John D. Rockefeller, American business magnate/philanthropist

195

There is always a way to go if you look for it.
-Ernest A. Fitzgerald, retired American Bishop of the United Methodist Church

196

You measure the size of the accomplishment by the obstacles you had to overcome to reach your goals.
-Booker T. Washington, African-American educator/author

197
There are risks and costs to a plan of action, but they are far less than the long-term risks and costs of comfortable in actions.
-John F Kennedy, 35th U.S. President

198
Successful men and women keep moving. They make mistakes, but they don't quit. **-Conrad Hilton, founder of the Hilton Hotels chain**

199
Remember happiness doesn't depend upon who you are or what you have; it depends solely on what you think.
-Dale Carnegie, American writer

200
When you cannot make up your mind which of two evenly balanced courses of action you should take - choose the bolder.
-William Joseph Slim, British military commander

201
Your life is in your hands, to make of it what you choose
-John Kehoe, lecturer

202
The most important key to achieving great success is to decide upon your goal and launch, get started, take action, move.
-John Wooden, American basketball coach

203

I think people who are creative are the luckiest people on earth. I know that there are no shortcuts, but you must keep your faith in something Greater than You, and keep doing what you love. Do what you love, and you will find the way to get it out to the world. **-Judy Collins, American singer, songwriter**

204

You can't have a better tomorrow if you are thinking about yesterday all the time. **-Charles F. Kettering, American inventor**

205

It is not how much we have, but how much we enjoy, that makes happiness.
-Charles Haddon Spurgeon, British preacher

206

Life is short, and it is here to be lived.
-Kate Winslet, actress

207

Learn from yesterday, live for today, hope for tomorrow. The important thing is not to stop questioning.
-Albert Einstein, German-born theoretical physicist

208
Anybody can do anything that he imagines.
-Henry Ford, American industrialist

209
It's your place in the world; it's your life. Go on and do all you can with it, and make it the life you want to live.
-Mae Jemison, American physician/NASA astronaut

210
Regret is an appalling waste of energy; you can't build on it; it's only good for wallowing in.
-Katherine Mansfield, writer

211
Your time on this earth is a gift to be used wisely. Don't squander your words or your thoughts. Consider that even the simplest actions you take for your lives matter beyond measure...and they matter forever.
-Andy Andrews, American author

212
You choose the life you live. If you don't like it, it's on you to change it because no one else is going to do it for you.
-Kim Kiyosaki, entrepreneur

213

Make sure your worst enemy doesn't live between your own two ears.
-Laird Hamilton, professional surfer

214

If you don't value your time, neither will others. Stop giving away your time and talents. Value what you know and start charging for it.
-Kim Grant, founder and CEO of a social media and personal branding company

215

Without goals and a plan to reach them, you are like a ship that has set sail with no destination.
-Fitzhugh Dodson, author/psychologist

216

Persistence can change failure into extraordinary achievement.
-Matt Biondi, former American swimmer

217

Pain is temporary. It may last a minute, or an hour, or a day, or a year, but eventually it will subside and something else will take its place. If I quit, however, it lasts forever. **-Lance Armstrong, retired American cyclist**

218
You've got to say, "I think that if I keep working at this and want it badly enough,I can have it." It's called perseverance.
-Lee Iacocca, American businessman

219
But you have to do what you dream of doing even while you're afraid.
-Arianna Huffington, Greek-American author

220
One of the most essential things you need to do for yourself is to choose a goal that is important to you. Perfection does not exist - you can always do better and you can always grow.
-Les Brown, motivational speaker and former politician

221
Continuous effort — not strength or intelligence — is the key to unlocking our potential. **-Liane Cardes, author**

222
Find a purpose in life so big it will challenge every capacity to be at your best.
-David O. McKay, author

223
Desire and imagination have the potential to position a person for greatness.
-Eric Thomas, motivational speaker/activist

224
Optimism is essential to achievement and it is also the foundation of courage and true progress.
-Lloyd Alexander, American author

225
Luck favors the mind that is prepared.
-Louis Pasteur, French chemist

226
The mind is the limit. As long as the mind can envision the fact that you can do something, you can do it, as long as you really believe 100%
-Arnold Schwarzenegger, bodybuilder/actor

227
Until you value yourself, you will not value your time. Until you value your time, you will not do anything with it.
-M. Scott Peck, American psychiatrist

228
Ability will never catch up with the demand for it.
-Malcolm Forbes, American entrepreneur

229
If you live long enough, you'll make mistakes. But if you learn from them, you'll be a better person. It's how you handle adversity, not how it affects you. The main thing is never quit, never quit, never quit.
-Bill Clinton, 42nd U.S. President

230
The first step toward success is taken when you refuse to be a captive of the environment in which you first find yourself.
-Mark Caine, American scientist

231
My best advice to entrepreneurs is this; forget about making mistakes, just do it.
-Ajaero Tony Martins, Nigerian entrepreneur/investor

232
Your success in life isn't based on your ability to simply change. It is based on your ability to change faster than your competition, customers and business.
-Mark Sanborn, author/speaker

233
Nurture your mind with great thoughts, for you will never go any higher than you think. **-Benjamin Disraeli, British Prime Minister**

234
The two most important days in your life are the day you are born and the day you find out why.
-Mark Twain, American author/humorist

235
Big goals get big results. No goals gets no results or somebody else's results. Every liability is just an asset in hiding.
-Mark Victor Hansen, American motivational speaker/author

236
Our intention creates our reality.
-Wayne Dyer, American self-help author

237
The biggest risk is not taking any risk. In a world that's changing really quickly, the only strategy that is guaranteed to fail is not taking risks.
-Mark Zuckerberg, founder of Facebook

238
Set your goals high, and don't stop till you get there.
-Bo Jackson, retired American baseball and football player

239
What's money? A man is a success if he gets up in the morning and goes to bed at night and in between does what he wants to do.
-Bob Dylan, American singer/songwriter

240
The vision of a champion is someone who is bent over, drenched in sweat, at the point of exhaustion, when no one else is watching.
-Anson Dorrance, American soccer coach

241
Do the thing you fear to do and keep on doing it... that is the quickest and surest way ever yet discovered to conquer fear.
-Dale Carnegie, American writer

242
What you become directly influences what you get.
-Jim Rohn, American entrepreneur

243
Don't limit yourself. Many people limit themselves to what they think they can do. You can go as far as your mind lets you. What you believe, remember, you can achieve.
-Mary Kay Ash, Mary Kay Cosmetics Founder

244
Passion is energy. Feel the power that comes from focusing on what excites you.
-Oprah Winfrey, American media proprietor/philanthropist

245
Enjoy the journey, enjoy ever moment, and quit worrying about winning and losing. **-Matt Biondi, former American swimmer**

246
You can only become truly accomplished at something you love. Don't make money your goal. Instead pursue the things you love doing and then do them so well that people can't take their eyes off of you.
-Maya Angelou, American author

247
Happiness depends upon ourselves.
-Aristotle, Greek philosopher

248
Nothing is impossible. With so many people saying it couldn't be done, all it takes is an imagination.
-Michael Phelps, multiple Olympic gold medalist (swimming)

249
Changing the big picture takes time.. and the best things to do is focus on the things that we can make in our lives if we're doing all that. That becomes the collage of real change.
-Michelle Obama, American lawyer/writer

250
Success is never permanent, and failure is never final.
-Mike Ditka, former American football player

251
Waste no tears over the griefs of yesterday.
-Euripides, tragedian of classical Athens

252
When one door of happiness closes, another opens, but often we look so long at the closed door that we do not see the one that has been opened for us.
-Helen Keller, American author, political activist, lecturer

253
If you judge people, you have no time to love them.
-Mother Teresa, Roman Catholic religious sister/missionary

254
Champions aren't made in the gyms. Champions are made from something they have deep inside them - a desire, a dream, a vision.
-Muhammed Ali, former American boxer

255
Nothing is impossible, the word itself says, "I'm possible!"
-Audrey Hepburn, British actress/humanitarian

256
I think that if you live long enough, you realize that so much of what happens in life is out of your control, but how you respond to it is in your control. That's what I try to remember.
-Hillary Clinton, politician

257
You can motivate by fear, and you can motivate by reward. But both those methods are only temporary. The only lasting thing is self motivation.
-Homer Rice, former American football player/coach

258
Whatever the mind of man can conceive and believe, it can achieve. Thoughts are things! And powerful things at that, when mixed with definiteness of purpose, and burning desire, can be translated into riches.
-Napoleon Hill, American author

259
Do not let the future be held hostage by the past.
-Neal A. Maxwell, apostle

260
When a goal matters enough to a person, that person will find a way to accomplish what at first seemed impossible.
-Nido Qubein, businessman and motivational speaker

261
To accomplish great things, we must not only act, but also dream, not only plan, but also believe.
-Anatole France, French novelist

262
Dream big and dare to fail.
-Norman Vaughan, American dogsled driver

263
I am not just here to make a living; I am here to make a life.
-Helice Bridges, Founder and CEO Difference Makers International

264
Things do not change, we do.
-Henry David Thoreau, American author

265
Be humble, be big in mind and soul, be kindly; you will like yourself that way and so will other people.
-Norman Vincent Peale, author/minister

266
Empower yourself and realize the importance of contributing to the world by living your talent. Work on what you love. You are responsible for the talent that has been entrusted to you.
-Catharina Bruns, founder of WorkIsNotaJob

267
Any man who selects a goal in life which can be fully achieved has already defined his own limitations.
-Cavett Robert, founder of the NSA (National Speakers Association)

268
Success consists of getting up just one more time than you fall.
-Oliver Goldsmith, Anglo-Irish novelist, playwright, poet

269
Anybody can do anything that he imagines.
-Henry Ford, American industrialist

270
A man is not finished when he is defeated. He is finished when he quits.
-Richard Nixon, 37th U.S. President

271
If you look at what you have in life, you'll always have more. If you look at what you don't have in life, you'll never have enough.
-Oprah   Winfrey,   American   media proprietor/philanthropist

272
If you don't have a dream, how are you going to make a dream come true?
-Oscar Hammerstein, lyricist and librettist

273
If you do things well, do them better. Be daring, be first, be different, be just.
-Anita Roddick, British businesswoman

274
Define success on your own terms, achieve it by your own rules, and build a life you're proud to live.
-Anne Sweeney, president of Walt Disney

275
Nobody's a natural. You work hard to get good and then work hard to get better.
-Paul Coffey, retired Canadian hockey player

276
You become what you think about.
-Earl Nightingale, English social reformer

277
The secret of joy in work is contained in one word – excellence. To know how to do something well is to enjoy it.
-Pearl S. Buck, American writer/novelist

278
In every success story, you will find someone who has made a courageous decision.
-Peter Drucker, American management consultant

279
The ability to learn faster than your competitors may be the only sustainable competitive advantage.
-Peter Senge, American systems scientist

280
You have to be open-minded when those early opportunities present themselves; take advantage of them whether they're going to make you a lot of money or not.
-Rachael Ray, American television personality

281
If something is important enough, even if the odds are against you, you should still do it. **-Elon Musk, South African-born, Canadian-American entrepreneur**

282
Make the most of yourself, for that is all there is of you.
-Ralph Waldo Emerson, 19th century American essayist

283
The more you love what you are doing, the more successful it will be for you.
-Jerry Gillies, American author

284
One chance is all you need.
-Jesse Owens, four-time Olympic gold medalist (track and field)

285
If you work just for money, you'll never make it, but if you love what you're doing and you always put the customer first, success will be yours.
-Ray Kroc, American businessman

286
The most difficult thing is the decision to act, the rest is merely tenacity.
-Amelia Earhart, American aviation pioneer

287
The fastest way to change yourself is to hang out with people who are already the way you want to be.
-Reid Hoffman, co-founder of LinkedIn

288
The best way of learning about anything is by doing.
-Richard Branson, English businessman

289
To be successful, you must act big, think big and talk big.
-Aristotle Onassis, business magnate

290
The road to Easy Street goes through the sewer.
-John Madden, football coach

291
Time is at once the most valuable and the most perishable of all our possessions.
-John Randolph, American politician

292
The surest way to not fail is to determine to succeed.
-Richard Brinsley Sheridan, Irish playwright

293
There is no failure only feedback.
-Robert Allen, American author/speaker

294
Fear begins to melt away when you begin to take action on a goal you really want. **-Robert G. Allen, author**

295
The great dividing line between success and failure can be expressed in five words: I did not have time.
-Franklin Field, author

296
Try not to become a person of success, but rather try to become a person of value.
-Albert Einstein, German-born theoretical physicist

297
The most splendid achievement of all is the constant striving to surpass yourself and to be worthy of your own approval.
-Denis Waitley, American motivational speaker

298
It takes less time to do a thing right than it does to explain why you did it wrong
-Henry W Longfellow, American poet/educator

299
There will never be another now. I will make the most of today. There will never be another me. I will make the most of myself.
-Robert H. Schuller, American Christian televangelist/author

300
You miss 100 percent of the shots you don't take.
-Wayne Gretzky, former hockey player

301
Have the end in mind and every day make sure you're working towards it.
-Ryan Allis, co-founder and CEO of iContact

302
Your aspirations are your possibilities.
-Samuel Johnson, English writer

303
The only disability in life is a bad attitude.
-Scott Hamilton, retired American figure skater

304
Always bear in mind that your own resolution to succeed is more important than any one thing.
-Abraham Lincoln, 16th U.S. President

305
The more willing you are to surrender to the energy within you, the more power can flow through you.
-Shakti Gawain, New Age author

306
Don't give up. There are too many nay-sayers out there who will try to discourage you.
Don't listen to them. The only one who can make you give up is yourself.
-Sidney Sheldon, American writer

307
Courage is the capacity to go from failure to failure without losing enthusiasm.
-Sir Winston Churchill, British politician, Prime Minister

308
The principle is competing against yourself. It's about self-improvement, about being better than you were the day before.
-Steve Young, retired American football player

309

Never underestimate the power of dreams and the influence of the human spirit. The potential for greatness lives within each of us.
-Wilma Rudolph, 3 time Olympic gold medalist (track and field)

310

Never let your failures go to your heart or your successes go to your head.
-Soichiro Honda, Japanese engineer/industrialist

311

Do not wish to be anything but what you are, and try to be that perfectly.
-St Francis de Sales, former Bishop of Geneva/honored as a saint in the Roman Catholic Church

312

Never give up on a dream just because of the time it will take to accomplish it. The time will pass anyway.
-Earl Nightingale, English social reformer

313

If you start to think the problem is 'out there,' stop yourself. That thought is the problem. **-Stephen Covey, American author**

314
Action may not bring happiness, but there is no happiness without action.
-William James, American philosopher/psychologist

315
You shouldn't focus on why you can't do something, which is what most people do. You should focus on why perhaps you can, and be one of the exceptions.
-Steve Case, co-founder of AOL

316
If you love what you do and are willing to do what it takes, it's within your reach. And it'll be worth every minute you spend alone at night, thinking and thinking about what it is you want to design or build.
-Steve Wozniak, American inventor

317
Be absolutely clear about who you are and what you stand for. Refuse to compromise. **-Brian Tracy, American author/motivational speaker**

318
Far and away the best prize that life has to offer is the chance to work hard at work worth doing.
-Theodore Roosevelt, 26th U.S. President

319
Your current situation is no indication of your ultimate potential!
-Anthony Robbins, life coach/self-help author

320
Anything is possible if you've got enough nerve.
-J. K. Rowling, pen name of British novelist

321
If we did the things we are capable of, we would astound ourselves.
-Thomas Edison, American inventor/businessman

322
You are the only real obstacle in your path to a fulfilling life.
-Les Brown, motivational speaker and former politician

323
You have to have your heart in the business and the business in your heart.
-Thomas J. Watson, American businessman

324
Even if something has just a one percent chance of success, success boils down to how fast you exhaust your ninety-nine failures.
-Thomas Jefferson, American Founding Father/3ʳᵈ U.S. President

325
Don't let what you cannot do interfere with what you can do.
-John Wooden, American basketball coach

326
Impossibility is an opinion, not a fact.
-Tom Landry, American football player/coach

327
Success is not final, failure is not fatal: it is the courage to continue that counts.
-Winston Churchill, former Prime Minister of the United Kingdom

328
The difference between the impossible and the possible lies in a man's determination. **-Tommy Lasorda, former baseball player**

329
Dream lofty dreams, and as you dream, so shall you become.
-James Allen, British philosophical writer

330

If you don't build your dream, someone will hire you to help build theirs.

-Tony Gaskins, motivational speaker

331

I do not believe in excuses. I believe in hard work as the prime solvent of life's problems.

-James Cash Penney, founder of the JC Penney stores

332

Chase the vision, not the money, the money will end up following you.

-Tony Hsieh, CEO and founder of Zappos

333

Our work is the presentation of our capabilities.

-Johann Wolfgang Von Goethe, German writer

334

Never dull your shine for somebody else.

-Tyra Banks, American television personality

335

Either write something worth reading or do something worth writing.

-Benjamin Franklin, author/diplomat

336
Never put an age limit on your dreams.
-Dara Torres, swimmer

337
If you have talent and you work long and hard at it, anything in the world can be yours. **-Unknown**

338
The price of success is hard work, dedication to the job at hand, and the determination that whether we win or lose, we have applied the best of ourselves to the task at hand.
-Vince Lombardi, head coach of the Green Bay Packers (1959-1967)

339
All of our dreams can come true if we have the courage to pursue them.
-Walt Disney, co-founder of the Walt Disney Company

340
If you don't think everyday is a great day, try going without one.
-Jim Evans, former major league baseball umpire

341
Mental attitude is more important than mental capacity.
-Walter Dill Scott, one of the first applied psychologists

342
Piling up material goods cannot fill the emptiness of lives which have no confidence or purpose.
-Jimmy Carter, Jr., 39th U.S. President

343
Work like there is someone working 24 hours a day to take it away from you.
-Mark Cuban, American businessman/investor

344
There is no scarcity of opportunity to make a living at what you love to do, there is only scarcity of resolve to make it happen.
-Wayne Dyer, American self-help author

345
The real challenge (in life) is to choose, hold, and operate through intelligent, uplifting, and fully empowering beliefs.
-Michael Sky, author

346
The price of excellence is discipline. The cost of mediocrity is disappointment.
-William Arthur Ward, author

347
Your work is going to fill a large part of your life, and the only way to be truly satisfied is to do what you believe is great work. And the only way to do great work is to love what you do.
-Steve Jobs, American entrepreneur/inventor

348
I hated every minute of training, but I said, "Don't quit. Suffer now and live the rest of your life as a champion.
-Muhammed Ali, former American boxer

349
Wake up every day knowing that today is a new day and only you can determine the outcome of that day. So dream big, accept the challenge, and never look back.
-Alicia Sacramone, retired American gymnast

350
Destiny is not a matter of chance; but a matter of choice. It is not a thing to be waited for. It is a thing to be achieved.
-William Jennings Bryan, politician

351
Nothing worthwhile comes easily. Work, continuous work and hard work, is the only way to accomplish results that last.
-Hamilton Holt, American educator

352
People inspire you or they drain you - pick them wisely.
-Hans F Hansen, retired soccer player

353
As long as one keeps searching, the answers come.
-Joan Baez, American folk singer/songwriter

354
Limitations live only in our minds. But if we use our imaginations, our possibilities become limitless.
-Jamie Paolinetti, cyclist

355
Show me a person who never made a mistake, and I will show you a person who never did anything.
-William Rosenberg, founder of Dunkin Donuts

356
May your future be worthy of your dreams.
-Barbara Bush, former First Lady

357
Don't wait until you feel like taking a positive action. Take the action and then you will feel like doing it.
-Zig Ziglar, American author/motivational speaker

358
If you want to be happy, set a goal that commands your thoughts, liberates your energy, and inspires your hopes.
-Andrew Carnegie, Scottish-American industrialist

359
It always seems impossible until it's done.
-Nelson Mandela

360
Do not watch the clock. Do what it does. Keep going.
-Sam Levenson, humorist

361
What you do today can improve all your tomorrows.
-Ralph Marston, football player

362
Motivation is what gets you started. Habit is what keeps you going.
-Jim Ryun, 1968 Olympic silver medalist (track and field)

363
At the end of the day, let there be no excuses, no explanations, no regrets.
-Steve Maraboli, bestselling author

364
First say to yourself what you would be; and then do what you have to do.
-Epictetus, Greek philosopher

365
Desire is the key to motivation, but it's determination and commitment to an unrelenting pursuit of your goal – a commitment to excellence – that will enable you to attain the success you seek.
-Mario Andretti, racing driver

Conclusion

I hope these quotes have inspired you as much as they've inspired me. I actually just filed for a second LLC today. If you would have told me 2 ½ years ago that I would own two different businesses, I probably wouldn't have believed you.

But remember, simply reading them does nothing unless you commit to putting them into practice! So now that you're armed with the motivation you need, put the book down, get out there, follow your dreams, and make your life amazing.

Lastly, THANK YOU for reading this book. If you would like to be notified of future publications, please click here and sign up for Kelli Rae's Publications Notifications. I will never share your information, and I will only send you an email when I have a new publication coming out.

If you would like to learn more about me or read any of my other publications, please visit my author page.

Resources
http://www.inspirational-quotes.info/
https://www.kabbage.com/blog/100-quotes-from-successful-entrepreneurs
http://www.forbes.com/sites/kevinkruse/2013/05/28/inspirational-quotes/
http://www.addicted2success.com
http://www.businessinsider.com/best-inspirational-quotes-from-us-presidents-2014-7
http://www.entrepreneur.com/article/233890
http://www.inc.com/peter-economy/21-inspiring-quotes-for-leaders.html
http://www.marieclaire.com/career-advice/tips/a11373/best-hillary-clinton-quotes/
http://www.businessinsider.com/inspirational-quotes-from-successful-people-2014-8
http://www.inc.com/jeff-haden/75-inspiring-motivational-quotes-for-being-happier.html
http://www.inc.com/jeff-haden/40-best-inspirational-quotes-for-entrepreneurs.html?cid=readmore

LASTLY - I want to say thank you for downloading my book and providing the support. I wish you the best in achieving your goals.

If you liked this bundle, I would appreciate any feedback. You can flip to the next page to leave a review on Amazon.

Again, thank you so much and have a super wonderful day!